Mastering the Art of Dominance

113 BDSM Troubleshooting Tips that Turn an Amateur into Expert Dom

Matthew Larocco

Copyright© 2017 by Matthew Larocco

Mastering the Art of Dominance

Copyright© 2017 Matthew Larocco
All Rights Reserved.

Warning: The unauthorized reproduction or distribution of this copyrighted work is illegal. No part of this book may be scanned, uploaded or distributed via internet or other means, electronic or print without the author's permission. Criminal copyright infringement without monetary gain is investigated by the FBI and is punishable by up to 5 years in federal prison and a fine of $250,000. (http://www.fbi.gov/ipr/). Please purchase only authorized electronic or print editions and do not participate in or encourage the electronic piracy of copyrighted material.

Publisher: Enlightened Publishing

ISBN-13: 978-1546905738

ISBN-10: 1546905731

Disclaimer

The Publisher has strived to be as accurate and complete as possible in the creation of this book. While all attempts have been made to verify information provided in this publication, the Publisher assumes no responsibility for errors, omissions, or contrary interpretation of the subject matter herein. Any perceived slights of specific persons, peoples, or organizations are unintentional.

This book is not intended for use as a source of legal, business, accounting or financial advice. All readers are advised to seek services of competent professionals in the legal, business, accounting, and finance fields.

The information in this book is not intended or implied to be a substitute for professional medical advice, diagnosis or treatment. All content contained in this book is for general information purposes only. Always consult your healthcare provider before carrying on any health program.

Table of Contents

Introduction 3

Chapter 1: The Mistakes Most Amateur Doms Make 7

Chapter 2: How Nice Guys Like You Can Turn Into a Better Dom 13

Chapter 3: Placing the Personal Ad 23

Chapter 4: Turning Your Friend with Benefits into a Sub 29

Chapter 5: How to Make a Good First Impression and Make a Friend 37

Chapter 6: A Good Way to Practice: Online Role Playing 45

Chapter 7: An Interview with a Successful Dom 49

Chapter 8: How to Help a Sub in a Downward Spiral 55

Chapter 9: Being a Friend First, a Dom Second 61

Chapter 10: How to Observe a Troubled Sub and Find Her Hidden Signals 73

Chapter 11: Creating a Therapeutic Curriculum to Build Self-Esteem 87

Chapter 12: Getting Professional Involved ... 95

Chapter 13: Working with Multiple Subs and Other Doms 101

Chapter 14: Dealing with Jealousy or Rivalries 113

Chapter 15: Parties, Threesomes, and Orgies with Multiple Subs 121

Conclusion 131

Other Books by Matthew Larocco 132

Introduction

Are you a frustrated Dom? Have you tried to be the best Dom possible but can't seem to find any subs? Do your sessions end prematurely? Are you not quite sure what you're doing wrong or how to start setting up programs for a sub that wants emotional healing?

You've come to the right place! Continuing our line of BDSM education books, we've compiled a list of tips that we call "Troubleshooting Tips", especially made for Doms who are stuck in a circle of inactivity.

Your subs may complain that you're too aggressive or too nice, or maybe that you just don't understand. The problem is not necessarily with you or your attitude. Usually it's because you haven't been formally trained on how to DIRECT a sub towards a progressive plan of action. It is your job to train a sub, explain the punishments and rewards, and transform her thinking.

You do have a tremendous responsibility set before you. No wonder most Doms flake out and decide the lifestyle is too complicated. Yes, if all you want to do is spank a few women or boys, or have NSA sex while wearing masks, then being a Dom isn't for you.

But if you want to help people grow, help people face their fears and overcome their flaws, and feel something cathartic and healing…then yes, you have a very worthy goal.

And if you've read my other books in the series, you have a good idea of where to start. Just because you haven't become the Dom you've always wanted to be in three easy steps doesn't mean it's impossible. You need a little more training and polishing.

No Dom has ever started off a complete natural. Everyone needs training and additional tips for turning their intermediate knowledge into professional / expert level understanding.

This book is going to teach you:

- How to attract subs (even if you've been unsuccessful in the past)

- How to avoid mentally disturbed subs before it's too late

- How to identify troubled subs who can be helped and how to help them

- How to manage multiple subs and multiple partners with fellow Doms

By the time you finish this book, you're going to be ready to be a top of your class Dom!

So, let's get started by discussing what you may be doing wrong...or at least, what 90 percent of all your peers are doing wrong.

Chapter 1: The Mistakes Most Amateur Doms Make

Most amateur Doms have a warped perspective of what discipline and submission entails, as they are being fed too much information on dominance and sadism, and not nearly enough on the psychology of submission.

Newcomers think that attitude is all it takes to be accepted into the lifestyle but it's more about knowledge. Most Doms come into a situation making the same mistakes:

- Having an aggressive attitude

- Displaying arrogance

- Using intimidation or bullying behavior

- Mistaking horniness for patience
- Being selfish when discipline actually requires great patience and compassion

As soon as you show yourself to be ignorant of the lifestyle, most potential subs will tune you out. You won't get replies. You will probably be insulted.

Consider some submissive-friendly tips on how to stop looking like an amateur.

#1: Rather than take offense and lash back at people who criticize you, try to learn from them.

Most people who are overly critical and downright rude can still do you the favor of explaining what you're doing wrong. You don't have to like the person or their attitude…but there's no sense in ignoring the good advice on how to improve. You can find many pearls of wisdom when others criticize your technique.

One of the first criticisms you will probably receive is:

#2: The Dom isn't always right. You don't have to be too proud to accept notes from a sub.

There may be some protocol to follow during a session. For example, a Dom saying that you have to give him a signal if you want to break character, or to wait until the session ends and you're both out of character before offering notes for improvement. But aside from breaking protocol, there is no golden rule that says the Dom cannot learn from the sub.

If the sub wants to suggest ways to improve safety, or technique, or just wants to try something different, a good Dom will take the counsel. Doms do make mistakes, especially in the beginning. If you establish a reputation as a Dom who doesn't negotiate, you will always be seen as an amateur.

Doms who defend their mistakes and try to blame the sub are just deluding themselves. Sometimes dominant behavior does go hand in hand with making final decisions and presenting yourself with full confidence. But if it's obvious that you messed up, the sub will lose respect for you if you don't take the responsibility for it.

Real Doms are strong enough to accept blame for what was clearly their fault and they are not going to try to shift the blame to someone else just to save face. A lot of macho guys think it's unmanly or submissive to admit that they made a mistake. Wrong! It shows honesty and strength to be able to humble one's self.

#3: Be picky. Don't settle for anyone less than someone you really like and are compatible with.

New subs will make the mistake of following anyone who calls himself Master or Dom. And it's too bad because they will be going home with a lot of losers who will only show them a bad experience. Masters and subs both should be picky about working with new people. Even if you're a level 0 and only want experience, resist going after the first sub you meet, just because they're available.

Spend a little time getting to know this person and what their limits and interests are. If there's something that seems off, or if you are opposites in some belief or kink, think twice about getting involved. Real Doms do not want to work with every single sub, nor should subs go home with just any Dom.

#4: You BOTH get pleasure from this experience. Not just you and not just her.

This is another mistake that a lot of newcomers make. Amateur Doms either think that their pleasure, their sadism, is all that matters, or the "Nice Guy Dom" is so intent on pleasing the sub, he doesn't actually give her the discipline she wants.

So no, you as the Dom are not obligated to pleasure every sub under the sun, as if you are at their beck and call. In fact, unless you both really enjoy each other's company, there's no good sense working in sessions where you are trying to please the sub but you don't actually enjoy any of the activities she's having you do. It's only natural to want to find someone who shares your interest, someone who deserves to meet your real personality and make use of your imagination.

#5: Don't rush into a relationship too soon.

BDSM activity is like sex in this way—far too many people just jump right into it without giving any serious thoughts to safety issues, emotional issues, compatibility issues and so on. Rushing into sessions is a mistake because it deemphasizes communication, trust and "learning" the other people. The more time you spend negotiating and sharing conversation beforehand, the less time you will spend apologizing or asking your sub to give you another chance.

These are common tidbits of advice given to new Doms that are making fools of themselves by coming on too strong, too early. In general, "be cool" and "don't try so hard" is what it boils down to. Don't be a psycho, an idiot, or a bully. Sounds simple enough, right?

However, there are actually many mistakes that even "smart Doms" make in the early stages and they can be tiring to a sub. Let's discuss some of these in the next chapter.

Chapter 2: How Nice Guys Like You Can Turn Into a Better Dom

Isn't the idea of a Nice Guy (the proverbial gentleman who ladies don't seem to like) disciplining a sub a paradox? Don't you have to be a little bit of an "asshole" to be able to punish a sub?

The truth is, no, it has nothing to do with that. While it's true that "nice guys" don't do well in dating, the reason is because they are ignorant—they don't know how to flirt or build attraction. The same is true in the BDSM lifestyle. Some Doms are so "nice" (or shall we say, ignorant as to what they're supposed to be doing) that they just end up boring subs rather than giving them the thrills they seek.

Some of the tips in this chapter are designed to turn you into a Thinking Dom, a cerebral lover, and not just a Dom with attitude.

#6: **Do not treat your sub like a sugar baby.**

BDSM is not a big daddy / sugar baby relationship. You are not here to spoil the sub. Too many Doms make the mistake of caving to the every desire of the sub, such as buying her toys, or doing just as she asks. In essence, when you surrender all control, the Dom has become the sex slave!

This only frustrates the sub or turns her into a brat, who will just manipulate you and eventually grow tired of you. This happens because:

1. You fall in love with your sub, which is not the intention of BDSM dating.

2. You don't really understand why she wants to be disciplined and submit.

3. She is not a good sub and is actually just a Dom wannabe playing you.

There could be other reasons, but those are the most common. Most subs will give you a chance and overlook a few errors. But if your discipline is non-existent, eventually they will realize that you're not a real Dom and you're more like a sub masquerading as a Dom, hoping to get lucky. Instead, it's very important to **train her**, as opposed to just giving her every good thing.

#7: When you give her what she wants, associate it as the natural reward of obeying you. She only gets what she wants when she pleases you.

You are now reversing the power dynamic. So yes, you will make her happy but only when she fulfills her duties as a **submissive party**. She will now feel as if she earned her reward, rather than just thinking of you as a pushover. An entitled sub is not submissive and so the dynamic is ruined.

#8: You must discipline…not just dominate.

Dominating someone is not the same thing as disciplining him or her. You can dominate someone because they let you, or because you're rough and strong, or because your personality is strong. However, disciplining someone involves training them to think and feel something—to teach them better behavior.

Some Doms are so intent on just dominating, (as screwing their subs' brains out) they don't ever think about disciplining them, teaching them, or guiding them to a new way of thinking or a new perspective.

Doms who never discipline show themselves to be weak. They may even allow their subs to break the rules, do half-hearted chores or forget to do something they were told to do. They may even break protocol or say something disrespectful.

You must discipline a sub when this happens!

Some Doms will literally just break the contract and stop seeing the sub if the sub has a disrespectful attitude. But some subs actually do just want to be punished for their behavior and so may subtly break the rules or bend them just to test your ability to discipline. So make them feel pain or rejection—in the manner in which you previously negotiated.

Subs thrive in relationships with boundaries and rules. Some Doms simply create reasons to discipline their subs, even if they are not rebelling. They may do this as a means of establishing control from the very beginning. As long as there is logic to their method, and it's organized as in a curriculum or timeline, then it's fine.

#9: Don't be a sadist. You must establish a reason for why you are punishing your sub, a system of rules that is established immediately.

You must set the rules and explain the consequences. They must clearly understand the expectations you have for them, so that they do have a chance to cooperate and be obedient.

#10: Punishment does not excite the sub. Punishment trains the sub.

Spanking a sub doesn't work if she enjoys being spanked. In this case, you would discipline her by actually removing some of her privileges and showing her that negative reactions have negative consequences.

Above all make sure she understands why she is being punished, and that the punishment fits the crime and doesn't take the training too far in terms of sadism.

#11: Remember that your rules are more important than the sub's pleasure.

This is a tricky concept to understand. Of course, the sub is the most powerful party and has the right to cease the arrangement if she so chooses. However, if a situation comes up where a sub breaks your rules by "accident" and not intentionally, then she still ought to be punished and not excused.

Why? Because your sub is not above your rules. Too many Doms make excuses for their subs and then inadvertently send them a message: that their training is pointless.

You must make the sub understand that she still answers to the rules, whosever rules they may be (yours in this instance) and that breaking rules demands punishment. So do not let negligence or ignorance slide. Give her corrective discipline and make sure she understands why she is being punished.

#12: Learn to Make a Damn Decision, Already!

Even outside of the BDSM lifestyle, women really get annoyed at a man that has no ideas and no suggestions on what to do. In BDSM, as a Dom, having a careless or deferring attitude is a major mistake!

Being indecisive paints you as weak and what she actually needs from you is great inner and outer strength. She is counting on you to make the BIG decisions and to micromanage her life (so as long as you are in each other's company). Some subs may even want you to exercise control over her, when she's not in your presence.

Remember that subs enjoy the feeling of surrendering all control. They may even be too stressed to make little decisions and so will count on you making these decisions for them.

This means you're going to have to start taking responsibility for your decisions, making educated decisions, and sticking by them.

And yes, if you make a mistake, you're going to have to admit it, fess up and move on. That's what being a dominant is all about.

#13: Remember the goal of soft limits and taboos: to gradually push them!

Hard limits are a definite "no crossing" and we've established that. But soft limits mean that the sub is attracted to the idea but still afraid of undergoing the experience. They may only give conditional consent, depending on the activity. Therefore, to bludgeon them with hardcore activities exploring their soft limit would be abuse of trust.

On the other hand, not slowly heading for that soft limit could be a major let down if the sub is hoping you will have the knowledge to slowly and comfortably explore the taboo.

The Taboo is really what you want to explore and if she's upfront about what she likes, your work is going to be easy. But if she is coy about what she wants and has a number of soft limits, then these soft limits would be the goal or "taboo" you're going to take on.

So you do want to push her limits but in a way where she is not afraid—where she is gradually eased into what she likes.

This is known as **growth** training.

#14: You must help your sub to GROW in the submissive process.

If she is already obedient to you from the start, then she doesn't grow. This is where your training and curriculum comes in.

Pushing your sub's limits and **expanding** her boundaries is the goal. This teaches her something new. You're giving her something for your sessions and the effort she put forth.

So while you do respect the limits, the failure to challenge her and teach her something **new** would be a disappointment in the long-run. The sub would not realize her full potential without a skilled teacher to bring this out of her. When a sub says that she has a soft limit she is not saying that she won't do it…just that she doesn't understand how she could be made to do it and not be afraid.

That's the challenge. For you to teach her how to enjoy the soft limit through a gradual process. This process would progressively move towards the soft limit as the goal.

More to the point, she will become bored. Too comfortable with the status quo and that is another mistake that most newcomer Doms make consistently.

#15: Create a curriculum based on the successful Dom "Growth Formula".

That is:

- Teach the sub why there is no reason to be afraid of the soft limit taboo.

- Teach the sub to be confident where she feels weak.

- Give the sub the experience she needs to undertake the soft limit.

- Help her understand what she's missing out on by creating a system of punishment and reward, based on activities that are related to the soft limit.

- Gradually expose her to the soft limit, one session at a time, in baby steps, and always according to each sub's individual needs.

Now granted, not all subs will be able to reach their soft limits and this is why you do have to stay attentive and stop the training if the sub becomes upset. If a sub can't even talk about an activity, then she may not be able to do it. You have to determine what she is ready for, what needs to be worked on, and whether she's capable of tackling these soft limits at all. She does have to have a desire to do something or else it is a **hard limit** and that mean no-go.

We'll talk more about more common Dom mistakes and ways to improve communication a little bit later. Thus far, you have a good idea on how to be an intermediate level Dom and how to stand out from a crowd of pretenders.

In the next few chapters, we're going to discuss how to go from intermediate Dom to an expert Dom—namely by finding your first real life sub!

Chapter 3: Placing the Personal Ad

First, understand that not many people are going to try to pick up strangers by saying "Hey, baby I'm a Dom." That just doesn't translate well outside of the lifestyle. Most of the people you meet that are willing to explore this kind of relationship are already familiar with the lifestyle. Even if you use a free site or a membership site, you're going to be putting in keywords related to BDSM, Dom, Sub, Discipline, Submission and so on.

The good news is that modern ads can be as long as you need, so you don't need to make it "short and sweet" since that's not going to establish any trust. When creating your dating profile, whether at sites like FetLife, Craigslist, Literotica, AdultFriendFinder or other popular alternative dating websites, keep the following tips in mind.

#16: Do not try to shock people with your Username. Choose something mysterious, interesting and very much "you".

Don't brag about your sexual prowess or size of any body part. Remember that BDSM is not always about sex. Broadcasting an embarrassing name and reputation is probably going to send the wrong impression about what you're looking for. Don't use your real name and only reveal information gradually, as you get to know a person.

#17: Try to avoid textspeak.

It's just not becoming of an intellectual conversation and may send mixed signals to subs who are looking for someone cerebral and strong-minded. Your goal is to come across as interesting, a little mysterious but with an overall "normal" disposition to show that you are trustworthy and the ideal Dom that a sub is looking for.

#18: Accentuate your positive qualities; reasons why a sub would love to have you.

The goal is not to brag and certainly not to lie. Rather to present the truth in a positive and interesting way. Excessive detail isn't necessary. In fact, some subs may be scared off by a Dom who writes too much.

Some of these positive qualities might include patience, an eagerness to please, the ability to cook, create products, a creative mind or musical talents. If the profile is exclusively for a BDSM community, you might also include other positives related to the lifestyle, such as knowledge of bondage and how to use rope, expensive toys, hosting in your home, and so on.

Once you compile all of your positive qualities, start writing sentences that explain these positives. You could even write about your negative traits, provided you speak of them in a positive manner, or use them to disqualify subs you do not want to work with. Sometimes subs may actually be attracted to you because you are dealing with the same negative traits that she is; for example, you're trying to quit smoking.

Another positive to include would be your association with SSC, RACK and PRICK, which means you understand the basics of the BDSM community and are a trustworthy person who takes standards and rules seriously. These association words mean:

- Safe, Sane and Consensual
- Risk Awareness Consensual Kink
- Personal Responsibility, Informed Consensual Kink

#19: Create another list for your ideal sub. Include the ideal match that you want to meet, as well as other types that you would still be willing to work with. Also include your hard limits and soft limits.

Now turn this into a series of additional sentences, making it clear who you are looking for and who you are not looking for. Whether it's a 24-7 slave, daddy dom, masochist, etc. you can make your desires known, thereby saving time by getting rid of the incompatibles.

#20: Include a face photo.

It's just smart thinking to rise to the top of the ranks by doing what others don't have the guts to do: put a profile picture. Close ups of your face or whole body shots in casual clothes work best.

Unless you want sexual BDSM encounters, don't include nude photos or sexual activity photos, as this would disqualify other subs who may not be interested in sex.

Don't give any personal information out as respects location, family or other personal details. The last thing you need is a stalker!

If you happen to be recognized by someone you know…well, that is a risk, but on the other hand, why is this friend or acquaintance searching a BDSM website anyway?

#21: When writing your ad, be likable, positive and humorous. Write about yourself and don't spend too much time discussing who you're looking for.

The goal of a dating ad is to "sell yourself". This means focusing on the incentive that the sub has for dating you. Be confident and don't use "sales language" or any form of dishonesty. Be specific when it comes to explaining your interests. Rather than say you like movies or going out to eat, list what movies and what meals you particularly like. You can also end the profile with a call to action, suggesting that anyone interested can talk to you.

If you don't seem to be getting any replies, then just rewrite the profile and make it a bit more exciting, funny or endearing. Shake things up, reword and experiment to see what gets the most responses.

It's fairly easy to start a conversation with a sub if you choose to communicate with strangers via the Internet. But other subs may want to use their BDSM knowledge to impress friends or lovers they already have. If that's the case with you, you're going to like the next chapter!

Chapter 4: Turning Your Friend with Benefits into a Sub

Working with strangers—someone you've met exclusively for BDSM—is much easier. You immediately establish the tone of the relationship and the power structure, as well as the energy between the two of you.

Friends with Benefits, Friends, BDSM partners, and serious lovers are all very different relationships with completely different "Rules." Therefore, if you want to turn one into the other, in this case a friends with benefit into a sub, you must focus on changing the relationship and introducing the "new rules" that will alter the existing dynamic. The same is true for turning anyone into your sub, whether that's a guy or girl that knows you as a friend, or a husband or wife, or a boyfriend and girlfriend.

The first step is to introduce the idea of BDSM as a casual conversation and not make a dramatic revelation about it. Think of introducing the conversation as a sort of "soft limit." Most people aren't opposed to it necessarily, they just don't understand it and do not know this aspect of your personality. So the project begins.

#22: Talk about what you've been reading or why you find it interesting on an intellectual level.

This is the introductory phase. You don't want to come on too strong by saying you want to try it with your friend/partner. You first want to test the waters. See how your friend or partner reacts and then evaluate how receptive they are to the idea.

They may be curious, perhaps laughing or smiling. Or maybe they would take offense, and if so, they would probably tell you why. If this is the case, you might find it useful to explain what real BDSM is and what misconceptions exist.

#23: The next step would be to broach the subject of you trying BDSM on your own. You might mention that you're looking for a partner. This immediately creates a visual in the other person's mind.

If they have a sexual interest in you already, as a significant other or as a friend with benefits, they might like the idea of casually experimenting with you. Most lovers are always ready to spice things up. The fact that you already want to do it will toy with their curiosity and may motivate them to volunteer.

If not, you can ask them directly and see if they have any objections to experimenting. Don't immediately say that you have a curriculum and do not act like a Dom right away. Right now the most important thing to do is establish trust.

#24: If you're not sexually active with the person yet, it will be more difficult. You must escape the friend zone by inciting the other person's jealousy.

Their primary defense against you is to not visualize you in any sexual way. Therefore, you can force them to experience sexual attraction to you, by discussing your sexuality in some way. This could be done by dating other people or talking about dating other people. If you think the other person can take it, and won't be frightened, you could even discuss your interest in BDSM, in erotic exploration, multiple orgasms, "subspace" and so on.

If there is any attraction at all, the idea of you with someone else will slowly pique at their minds. Exhibiting the qualities that they find attractive, as well as a dominant attitude, will also help.

After a period of time, you could try stating your feelings for the friend to see if this sparks any curiosity in the friend. But don't get your hopes up. Breaking out of the friend zone is not always an easy process and it requires the right circumstances, where you can spend time with them and seduce them through casual conversation.

They key is in changing the dynamic and separating yourself from them, showing them that until they can accept you as a lover, you cannot be friends anymore. Essentially, you play the Dom Daddy and punish your friend for not giving you the romantic attention you crave. This tactic doesn't work 100% of the time but it's a good place to start.

#25: Determine each other's hard and soft limits.

You don't have to do this "officially" if this is still a hypothetical conversation. Make it fun or casual; Truth or Dare, or just a list of things the other person has thought about doing, or has done in the past. This is a way of drawing the other person out and making them reveal their desires.

Pay attention to their hard limits and soft limits. If they confess something they've always thought about trying but never have because of nervousness, this is a soft limit you can explore.

All that's left now is to offer to be the Dom and officially start the contract and negotiation process.

#26: Don't neglect any of the process just because you're friends or partners. In fact, it's doubly important to retain trust and not allow for any misunderstandings.

The last thing you need is to ruin the friendship in addition to ruining the BDSM session. Communicate, be kind and gradually introduce the scene.

#27: Take the relationships slower. Plan more sessions with less severe or challenging activity.

Because you're dealing with a friend, you really have to take it at a slower pace so that you can build more trust as a lover and guardian before trying to train or discipline the friend.

The friend is usually not going to challenge you, at least at first. So don't go heavy on the discipline. Focus on becoming a dominant presence, and breaking away from the "friend" mode in which you treat each other as equals. If she agrees to this arrangement, she must become submissive to you. Gradually, your friend may even test you by being uncooperative with your training. This means you must punish her, or if she doesn't cooperate after that, end the kinky relationship.

This is why some friendships simply cannot survive a BDSM experiment. Be aware of this and if you sense the friendship is becoming endangered cease all discipline-related activity. At some point, if the experiment fails you must decide that the friendship is more important to keep than the BDSM arrangement.

Now that we've established the initial conversation, let's move on to discussing how to keep the positive attitude going and make a new sub receptive to your offer.

Chapter 5: How to Make a Good First Impression and Make a Friend

First impressions mean everything and particularly in BDSM, since that first encounter establishes the energy of the entire relationship. You screw up here, it's going to be very difficult to gain back that respect and trust.

This section is divided into two parts: making a new relationship with a sub individually as well as making a good impression at a party. Let's start with the individual sub.

#28: Always be respectful and kind for an introduction.

Do not have an attitude and definitely avoid being "in character." You're not playing yet so don't act like anything other than yourself. You or the sub can start with an introduction.

Don't be giggly, nervous or affable. The projection of confidence and success is very important. So yes, you are ideally a little bit restrained. However, that doesn't mean you compromise your alpha qualities. Be strong and simply be welcoming to a newcomer.

#29: Just because you're talking to a new sub doesn't mean you're going home with him/her.

Be "friends" first and don't jump into a BDSM psychosexual state yet. You're not the Dom Daddy and she's not the bad girl. You're just two people meeting each other and learning the **peripherals** first.

If the sub shows ignorance, (such as calling you Master without knowing you) do not take her home. You don't have to be rude about it, but you should explain (preferably in private) that no sub should show this respect to someone they don't yet know. Explain that the Dom needs to earn the sub's respect. Maybe the sub will appreciate the lesson and try to work with you later on.

#30: Sir or Ma'am will suffice. Do not demand subs call you anything while you're out of character and just introducing yourself.

Once the both of you are comfortable you can start discussing contracts, negotiations, hard and soft limits, kinks and the like.

Remember the game doesn't actually begin until the session. The negotiation phase is typically out of character, as is the aftercare. However, it is essential that you always maintain your confidence. Do not show your weakness. Do not instantly defer to the sub even out of character. Be proud of who you are and always look and sound professional.

Group Settings

In group settings, the dynamic is similar. Be friendly and polite. Address people as sir or ma'am, or by their name and not in character. Don't be alarmed if some subs say something like: "Hello Sir, I'm Amanda, and I belong to Jake. Nice to meet you." These subs are ordered to make their ownership known, so as to remind you that she is not available, or at least not without permission from her Dom.

Munches are group events where everyone gathers in a "vanilla" location and mainly stay out of character, though they sometimes chat about kinks. However, the main intent is to simply be normal and meet new people in the community.

#31: Be outgoing and friendly.

Some Doms make the mistake of separating themselves from the group, which sends body language suggesting that they do not want to be approached. Not only should you be friendly but being a little more outgoing than usual will always help you. If you keep to yourself, especially as a Dom, you will look suspicious. So right away they think that you are either nervous, or snotty, or even creepy.

#32: Always make eye contact and talk about positive things.

Running out of things to say and going back into your shell is a bad first impression. So many new Doms do not make eye contact but remain off to the sidelines. That doesn't say much about their confidence, does it?

Don't just answer questions with yes or no. Put thought into your answers. Rehearse a few sentences in case the other people at the munch run out of things to say. Remember, you don't have to talk about sex or BDSM play at all. Just show them you're a normal, sane and knowledgeable person.

#33: When the group does something, make an effort to go be near them, sit with them, and contribute to the conversation.

It may feel like ingratiating yourself, but as long as you don't interrupt anyone, they won't mind!

Most groups are receptive to new people and the new energy they bring to the group. Obviously, you don't want to say anything controversial. You don't want to brag or talk about sex gratuitously. If there's a funny story or a casual mentioning of BDSM activity, it should be okay. Be mature and always speak with class. Look classy and dress well.

#34: If you attend a BDSM event or a "High Protocol / Play Party" understand that everyone is sort of in character. Do your best to fit in and show respect.

These parties simply demonstrate to you some of the BDSM activity that the community enjoys. However, it is not an orgy and there are always rules that must be abided by. Pay attention to any notices about dress code or conversation.

Most of the BDSM play will be just for you to watch and not participate in. You are never required to watch if the scene makes you uncomfortable. But there's no need to make a scene or judge anyone. Never touch anyone without permission, nor their belongings. Do not do anything that would be considered inappropriate in the outside world, such as taking unauthorized photos or video footage.

Don't be rude to any staff members or any subs. Only the Dom has the right to discipline their sub(s).

If you are talking to another Dom it is considered polite to not introduce yourself to his sub but to wait until the Dom introduces her to you.

#35: After you meet a friendly sub that seems to be interested, slow things down.

It is often suggested in the BDSM community that you not immediately go home with or host somebody you just met. It's a risk, and contrary to popular belief, just because you meet someone on an online forum or a munch, doesn't mean it's safe to go home with them!

It's up to you to establish trust over time. Talk on the phone, through email and arrange for a few in-public dates that do not involve any play. There is no rush. You can always count this as the negotiation process. There's simply no need to jump into a scene.

If something about the other person seems off, then just listen to your instincts and postpone going home with them. It's not wise to take a chance, believing that everyone in the BDSM community is a nice and trustworthy sub/Dom. Don't make any decision to plan scene until you feel safe in their presence and until you have negotiated everything.

#36: When you do finally stage a scene and a location, arrive separately. One of you leaves early.

This is the standard protocol and is often suggested to subs by Doms so that they can feel safe. You do not need to know where the sub lives or what kind of car they drive, so do not insist upon this. If and when the sub feels comfortable telling you, then you can know.

#37: Tell someone where you're going and arrange for them to call you if you do not text them at a reasonable time. Tell the sub to do the same thing. It creates responsibility and also protects the both of you.

Simply put, create your own list of rules to follow, and for the sub to follow, that will increase her trust in you. If she doesn't like your set of rules then move on. You must feel comfortable in this setting if you are to thrive, just the same as the sub.

In the next chapter, we will discuss another safe scenario worth investigating. The online role play!

Chapter 6: A Good Way to Practice: Online Role Playing

Online role-playing is a great way to gain experience for novices and intermediates. It's also a great way to improve your communication skills while waiting to meet someone else in person. Online role playing can sharpen your imagination as people do seem to share more willingly when only speaking in text.

You can become more immersed in a scene, considering that you don't have physical limitations inhibiting you. You can add accompanying music, porn images or other stimuli that helps you visualize the action, allowing you type and write more vividly.

There are many online role playing forums and websites where you can connect with other role players to tell a story. If you are a man you may have to be a little persistent since most online erotic role players are men. If you are a woman you may have to be a little open-minded and choose the most imaginative offer, which will be one out of about 1000!

#38: You might find better success if you create a scenario or a "theme" that you work with the most.

Players might find this intriguing, whether it's a special kink (Boss and employee, mother and stepson, etc.) or if it's erotic fanfiction of an existing series/movie. You may get more offers this way. The more experience you rack up in role playing this particular kink the more expertise you can bring to in-person sessions.

#39: Be polite and imaginative in your profile.

It seems to be difficult to be both but it can be done. A lot of role players get overly excited and take on an aggressively sexual and selfish tone which many genuine subs find off-putting. The best way to find a real partner on an online forum is to create a detailed profile, with either your picture or a picture that corresponds to your niche. Someone may find your profile interesting and start discussing fetishes to see if there is compatibility.

#40: If you're secure in your sexuality, pretend to be an opposite gender and test your imagination.

While frowned upon in real life dating, live text role playing as the opposite gender can be a good practice for enhancing your vocabulary and erotic imagination. It can help you learn what it's like to be the opposite gender sub, and see where so many other Doms go wrong.

You will definitely get a lot of poor quality Doms offering to virtual punish you. Pay attention and you can learn from their mistakes. Take notes and determine how you would handle the role play differently.

Do not use lazy "text speak". Take the time to type all the words out, as if writing an article or story.

When you're ready, find an opposite sex sub that really does match you and start a normal conversation that eventually leads into cyber BDSM play.

#41: You could and should turn this online fling into a more intimate relationship when the time is right.

You could follow up a few online BDSM role plays with a phone conversation, or a video chat. Eventually, you could even travel to meet this person and perform the role play scenarios in person.

In the next chapter, we're going to interview a real life Dom and get some answers to commonly asked questions. You're going to like the bluntness and honesty of our special guest, especially when it comes to motivating new Doms.

Chapter 7: An Interview with a Successful Dom

Our Dom chose for anonymity but he comes from a background of BDSM certification and a skill set that includes role play, bondage, discipline and hosting parties after dark. For this chapter, we'll be having a Q & A with Mister Black.

Q: What have you found searching sites like Tinder and Craigslist?

MB: It's really a gamble when you use free sites or non-niche sites. You may occasionally find the real deal; a Dom or a couple of swingers. But a lot of times you find people with major issues, jealousies and psychoses. I would recommend a BDSM website that is well reputed and trafficked. Like *FetLife* or an online role play community like *HumanPets* or *Sociolotron*. Even *Second Life* is a great place to meet people when you're just starting out. But when it comes to time to find a real partner I would look up MUNCH parties at local hangouts. It's just better practice to learn who people are in real life rather than always meeting them "in character."

Q: What do most Doms do wrong when they're just starting out?

MB: Finding someone that doesn't match them. True, there are some idiots out there that don't understand discipline at all. But more often than not the Dom has good intentions…he just can't find the right match. So he's either too aggressive or too soft. More time should be spent making friends and getting to know people. Once you find a good friend you can take the time to discuss likes and dislikes in the negotiation. Overall, spending more time search will help improve your odds.

Q: What is the best pick up line for a Dom looking for a sub?

MB: Don't use one liners! So many Doms online and even in person just think one line is going to find them a great sex life. But it's really about what you can say that's going to show the sub you have value; that her time will not be wasted with you. The sub wants something in exchange for your pleasure. Think in terms of what you, the Dom, can bring to the sub. What's the incentive? Of course, you don't start a conversation with a promise. You start a conversation like a man, or at least in my case I do! If you really need advice on how to talk like a man, watch some old school Hollywood movies from the 1940s and 1950s. I like Clark Gable myself. He had great eye contact, great voice and I always liked the way he worded sentences.

Q: Why do a lot of relationships end prematurely after they begin?

MB: In my case it's because the sub just doesn't understand the dynamic and makes no effort to try and improve. If I can see that she's not serious and is just looking to create drama, I end the relationship by the second session. My time is valuable in this [BDSM] lifestyle and outside of it. For Doms, I'd say probably because they don't have direction on where they're going. They haven't really thought the relationship through in terms of what am I really teaching her, what am I showing her? They just think Discipline is all about spanking a girl and that's not what it is.

Q: What tips can you provide about getting your sub to subspace?

MB: Mostly intimacy and not just aggressive punishment. I always say it's a side effect of love, not just physical action. She has to see you as a rock, as an authority figure that communicates love. If you don't have that trust, it's going to be an awful experience. When I first started in the lifestyle, I had a Domme who really didn't know what she was doing. She just whipped me for minutes on end and it hurt. I guess she thought I just enjoyed getting spanked…which I did. But what I really wanted at that time in my life was someone to trust. Eventually I just stopped going because I felt no love or intimacy from the experience, and that's why we do it—that's the whole point.

Q: What advice do you have for a Dom who isn't quite getting the hang of it and can't find a long-term sub?

MB: Spend more time working on yourself. If subs don't like you it's because you're trying too hard, but not focusing on yourself. Your positive qualities. You must let those shine. She should feel great warmth and great authority coming from you. Meditate more. Focus on what turns you on more. Find ways to incorporate your natural talents into role play and the scenes. The better you are as a man and a human being, the better of a Dom you will be. Attitude is nothing…an experienced sub can feel your heart, you know?

Chapter 8: How to Help a Sub in a Downward Spiral

Of course, it's not ideal that you should be a person's therapist. You are not a trained medical professional and you are not obligated to save someone who is determined to do stupid things and suffer from their own poor decisions. This is the "downward spiral" we all know and fear.

Then again, turning your back on someone who obviously needs help is hard to do. It's heartbreaking to watch. So even though it's less than ideal, you are going to have to play an unofficial therapist...just long enough to help your sub back up and on two feet again. While the ultimate goal is to have someone else look after the ailing sub, very often that is not an option. The sub may not even want to go get help from anyone else, except maybe you.

That means you are not only a Dom, and a friend, but now acting as a therapist, hoping to steer the sub in a positive direction. If you're going to do this (once again, you don't have to!) don't take the assignment lightly.

Here are some basics to remember:

1. Your sub is suffering from low self-esteem. You must build her back up.

2. Your sub doesn't need to be humiliated or browbeaten. They are already feeling at their lowest ebb.

3. They do need strong discipline.

4. You need to have a goal in mind for them, with every session.

5. Consider rehabilitation your goal, not just sexual or kinky motivations.

6. Do not attempt to become a doctor or therapist and "cure them". That's not your job.

#42: Understand that most subs in a downward spiral are either in denial of their behavior, are unaware of what they're doing, or are afraid of being "labeled" as mentally incompetent. Do not sound overly critical. Do not sound as if you are questioning their ability to run their own lives.

You CAN express concern about them. However, if you want the conversation to stay positive you must avoid sounding judgmental. Do not be insensitive and say something like "Snap out of it" or "it's all going to be okay."

#43: Allow the sub to vent but only when she is ready.

The sub may not want to talk AT ALL for the first few sessions. They know exactly what they want from you, and it may be sexual, or it may involve spankings, or other roleplays. They are requesting these things for a reason; perhaps as a distraction from their own thoughts or maybe even as preliminary actions to confronting the painful truth.

You are not going to force the sub to talk, but let them know they can always confide in you, ether in session or out of session, or "character." Sometimes it's better to vent outside of a session or scene, just as two human beings.

#44: You can reward the sub or discipline the sub in the ways they find appropriate. You don't have to force them to confront their demons before they're ready.

Give them the sex, spanking or other punishment they want. Do not let them challenge you or disrespect you. You must establish control and let them know you are not a push over. They cannot take their anger out on you. Not if you're going to be their Dom. Establish yourself as an authority figure.

#45: Give them a pep talk and build their self-esteem, in character and out of character.

A system of reward in this case, would not only be sexual or kinky behavior, but also discussions where you build the sub's self-esteem up. Do not give them praise for nothing. Make them earn it. They earn your inspiring talk by obeying your commands.

In theory, subs in a downward spiral want to suffer. They want their reward, but they also crave discipline from someone stronger than they are. Therefore, one of the crucial lessons you will teach them is that there are consequences for every action.

#46: Do not reward bad behavior. Do not give them anything in pity.

Rebellious children, and yes even the self-destructive "adult children" you sometimes meet in life, must not be allowed to get away with anything. No matter their manipulations or begging.

We punish our friends even outside of the BDSM lifestyle, even though we don't realize it. We cut off money from people who waste it. We cut off association with friends who are becoming abusive. We are in essence training them on the way they ought to behave when around us.

The same is true within a BDSM context. When subs act out, you as the Dom punish them. Not by giving them pleasure but by removing something they like. Or by inflicting a level of agreed upon pain.

#47: If you "break them", be kind and compassionate. Instruct them on what they need to do next.

You're not trying to "break them" by any means. But after punishment, and perhaps after a reward of inspirational talk, the sub may start crying. Proceed to aftercare immediately and cease being in character.

You can still be confident, dominant and authoritative. But now your voice must be calm and reassuring. You must communicate love and concern. You are not excusing their wayward course of life but want to encourage them to find productive solutions.

Resist crying or becoming angry or anything that feels like desperation. You have to be strong right now because they want to lean on you.

Aftercare is not the time for punishment. This is a time for healing and as you remember from the aftercare discussion in our other line of books, aftercare is a time of tenderness, holding, caressing, touching and talking.

If the sub is in a desperate state, as with drug addiction or something else that could turn fatal, it is essential that you guide them to professional help as quickly as possible. This will be the subject of a later chapter.

In the meantime, let's discuss some specific ways that you can be a friendly and helpful Dom, even when the sub is falling apart.

Chapter 9: Being a Friend First, a Dom Second

Simply put, a bad Dom is a bad friend. A bad friend makes a bad Dom. What it all comes down to is that a Dom is a sub's friend and wants to help the sub improve herself and experience the closure she needs to move on with her life. If a sub is on a downward spiral and engaging in self-destructive behaviors, then she is more in need of a friend than just a good time.

#48: Do not lecture the sub too early on. She hasn't earned your wisdom or guidance yet. If she claims she just wants to have fun, arrange to meet and show her a good time. Lure her in and then surprise her with a life lesson later on.

No sub is going to cooperate if you try to lecture her in advance and guilt trip her before a relationship starts. Make her feel comfortable. Make her feel welcomed and without any judgment. This process should be about earning her trust and nothing more. Let her know that although you do have your rules, this relationship is also about her getting what she wants. (Not what she "needs"…that comes later) But the only way that happens is if she becomes submissive to you.

#49: Exercise caution when it comes to trusting strangers…especially ones who appear to be dangerous.

Remember what we said earlier about trusting people too soon. Do not feel pressured to take her home with you or meet in any location just because she seems desperate. Only go when you feel comfortable. Limit your meetings to public places until you feel comfortable. If the issue of security bothers you, create a protocol where she is always at your mercy and trusting you, and not the other way around.

Be a Big Brother Dom

Of course, part of being a good Dom is simply learning how to improve yourself as a good friend. These next tips are suggestions on how to improve the quality of work you do, by increasing your attentiveness and committing yourself to a sub in a spirit of love and a sincere desire to help.

#50: Make your new relationship a committed one.

This not only means to stop seeing other subs temporarily, but also to keep your promises and devote yourself fully to her recovery. Take all your commitments seriously. Just because you're the Dom doesn't mean that you can arbitrarily decide to cancel sessions or arrive late. This is considered rude behavior and paints you in a poor light.

#51: Do not be afraid to say NO.

This is a major problem with new Doms and it's even worse when you have a self-destructive sub. Never give in to the sub's manipulation and give her what she wants, without her first earning it. This may require you to say no quite a bit, whether for her learning experience or your comfort.

Even Daddy Doms do not spoil their princesses and give them everything they want. She is not in a position to decide what she needs—you are. She needs guidance, not luxury. She cannot make good decisions on her own until you teach her how to do that.

Even if she cries, do not give in. It doesn't matter whether she's faking or legitimately crying because you're denying her something she asked for. She cannot break the rules and get a reward. That's not how it works. It is your job to protect and care for her and her job to obey. Saying NO is a form of discipline. She needs discipline right now. You are not a bully, but a loving big brother.

#52: Make notes of all the important things.

The sub really needs to feel as if she is important to you and she is. A good Dom doesn't abuse a sub by suggesting she's unwanted. Instead, he takes notes of every important item in the sub's life, whether it be names, dates, favorite snacks and foods, lovemaking positions, favorite colors, family life (if requested) and other information. Always make it a priority to remember these things. Reminding her that you really know her, appreciate her, and take these things seriously will quickly establish trust.

When she confides in you information it is a sign of great trust.

#53: Always make her the center of attention.

Attention is what she needs the most right now. Allowing anything else to distract you will send a mixed message. Your sub WILL grow increasingly obsessed with you, but so long as she respects the rules, this can be to her benefit.

Once she gets the privilege of spending time with you, take that time seriously. Make her feel like she's the center of attention. Turn off all cell phones and do not allow any other interruptions, whether it's work, family or friends.

You can also send her little "rewards" (if she merits them) by sending her texts, emails, letters or phone messages from your home or job. If she talks to you on the phone or chat, resist "surfing around" or dividing attention.

#54: Do not check out other subs in her presence.

Men especially have a problem with this. And while this differs among various types of subs, when you are playing big brother Dom to a destructive sub, checking out other people and being distracted by them is a hard blow to a person's self-esteem. The sub is hyper sensitive and feeling quite jealous. Until you can help her to build self-esteem you should not be caught eyeing other women or giving anyone else your attention.

#55: Always keep your promises.

This is not negotiable because the sub is counting on you to fulfill your promises. So that means, first of all, you don't promise anything you cannot ensure. You take seriously everything you say you're going to do and follow through on it.

Granted, sometimes meeting obligations may be impossible, due to emergency situations and the like. This doesn't mean the promise is broken. Simply explain to the sub that something came up but that you will still give her what you said as soon as another opportunity rises. She may feel disappointed at first, but showing her that you are determined to keep your word will go a long way in building trust.

If you break promises constantly and are always disappointing her, you are not only a bad Dom but also further hurting her self-esteem.

Remember that your submissive's greatest desire is to feel valued and important in your life. She needs reassurance and she will work hard to earn your compliments, rewards and praise. Being a Dom of your word is crucial especially at this stage.

#56: Don't just promise…show. Be a good example.

While disciplining and praising the sub, you will be creating tasks for her to accomplish. They should be challenging but doable. Not too easy but certainly not impossible. In order to be truly effective, these tasks should be something that you can do. The reason being a good example from you will go a long way in making the sub want to work harder. Giving the sub a course on how to be more like the Dom (and take on those better qualities that will build her self-esteem) is a great way to give the curriculum a feeling of productivity.

On the other hand, if you demonstrate a bad example, the sub will lose all motivation. On certain days, you may not feel like disciplining or being dominant with your sub and she may not feel very submissive. But if you approach the situation with low energy, she will quickly imitate you and only give half-hearted responses.

You must lead by example. You must live up to your responsibilities to her. Your actions will always speak louder than your words: If you don't, your sub will gradually start breaking the rules and may eventually stop responding to discipline. If that's the case, the relationship is doomed…and right when she needed you most!

#57: **Never keep any secrets.**

Now this doesn't mean that the Dom allows the sub to be nosey and interfere in business that's not hers. It simply means that a Dom cannot afford to make a mistake when it comes to keeping secrets or lying to the sub.

If he is not being exclusive with her, make this known upfront. If the sub needs full attention for the time being, then give it to her…but always with the knowledge that this will be temporary. Simply put, the more secrets you keep, the worse it's going to turn out if the sub thinks you've been deceiving her.

Quite frankly, unhinged subs who feel betrayed can get violent! So always be upfront about something, even if it's not pleasant news. It's much better to say it at the outset then try to hide secrets later on…and get busted.

Subs can be very nosey, and especially when they sense you are keeping a secret. They need reassurance constantly and if you are being elusive or mysterious, it's basically a punishment to them! They will rebel and maybe even go through your things.

If they don't find anything, and if you have stayed true to your word, it will be time to discipline the sub. But most importantly, she will trust you even more so. Because she will see that you are an open book and have nothing to hide. And yes, you really do love her that much, that you have no secrets.

Some Doms even give their passwords to the sub as a reward, as in "you can check in on me if you get worried." It's not a move of deference, but the move of a dominant parental figure who knows the sub is feeling anxious.

#58: Establish limits early on…and mean it!

It is especially important when training a self-destructive sub to set limits on how long the relationship will last, and indeed, how long until you encourage the sub to seek professional help. Otherwise, the sub may eventually fall in love with you and may want something from you that you cannot provide.

If you go exclusive with a sub who begins to NEED you, that relationship could evolve into a master-slave relationship.

Are you ready for that kind of commitment? If you are, then that's a tremendous responsibility and one that you cannot just walk away from. It's cruel to toy with a sub's emotions and promise her something that you cannot live up to.

In fact, it's not recommended that you go back to a vanilla "equality" based relationship with a sub after you've started a Dom-sub relationship. By choosing this lifestyle you establish rules and expectations for each other. To suddenly break those rules is a huge risk. This is why it is actually difficult to turn a "friend" into a sub. It really is two different worlds colliding.

Ownership of a slave is a responsibility much like taking in a "grownup child". You must protect and nurture her, as a wife, but with the added responsibility of discipline and love. The power dynamic must stay intact as that will define the relationship. You may even have to sacrifice some of your own wants for the sub's needs.

So if you don't want a fully devoted sub, you MUST establish when the relationship should end and stick to it. Make no secret that the relationship is finite and CANNOT go on indefinitely. Even if you don't establish a date, the end of the relationship must be discussed. You have to concentrate on teaching her a new authority besides you. Namely, herself, her family and friends, and the professional help she needs to get her life back on track.

You owe her this much. You need an exit strategy that will not leave her feeling alone or abandoned. You owe her closure. Once again, you must be a man of your word and one with no secrets.

In the next chapter, we're going to discuss the warning signs and red flags that the sub you're meeting may be emotionally unbalanced and potentially dangerous. What you decide to do once you know is your prerogative, but learning what to look for is essential.

Chapter 10: How to Observe a Troubled Sub and Find Her Hidden Signals

To some extent, you want to avoid troubled subs. On the other hand, you might someday meet a sub who is troubled but still relatively sane. Perhaps this is a person you might want to work with, after taking some time to learn who they are.

In this chapter we're going to discuss two groups of behaviors of subs; one that points to insane, and not worth befriending, and the other that indicates "troubled" but not necessarily unfit for a relationship.

#59: Any sub that acts like a Dom is obviously bad news.

The role of the sub is to be submissive or at least cooperative, so that she can be made submissive. If the sub is aggressive and giving you orders then they're a Dom or maybe a switch, approaching you the wrong way. Switches should not force Doms to be subs if that's not what they're looking for. Be wary of anyone who doesn't understand proper BDSM play.

#60: Avoid anyone in the community or out that exhibits psychotic behavior.

Subs are warned to stay away from Doms who are being emotionally manipulative and the same is true for Doms who are on the lookout for subs. Pay attention to how these emotionally unstable people make you feel.

Dangerous or insane people will:

- Use fear or intimidation to force you into a relationship

- Threaten to leave you in hopes of extorting loyalty

- Threaten violence if you don't cooperate

- Ignore your needs or basic safety protocols

- Question your loyalty or become unhinged if you question their behavior (especially in aftercare or negotiation)

- Bribe you with expensive gifts to get you to do something you don't want to do

- Make you feel unattractive or unwanted

- Make you feel guilty if you do not want to do something

- Toy with crossing your hard limits

- Make you feel afraid to end the relationship because of their reaction

Some subs are actually very aggressive people and they really like to bully other Doms and subs. They may submit to their Doms, but they may actually just enjoy toying with others like you. Don't give them the time of day.

If you have explained the natural end to the relationship in advance, there should not be a problem. But if the sub seems unwilling to let the relationship go this could definitely be a red flag.

#61: Beware of subs with exaggerated emotions.

While BDSM is about summoning intense emotion, which is the reward of a good scene, when a sub enters into a relationship already exaggerating her reactions or emotions, this is usually a red flag showing that the sub may be insane or at least very hard to handle.

Intelligent, mature and rational subs can keep their emotions under control until they allow themselves to "release" under a good Dom. Emotional responses occur when an individual feels that they are beyond controlling. Highly emotional subs at the very beginning of the relationship demonstrate their instability by showing explosive anger, out of control optimism and a sort of "all over the place" personality.

You may be able to work with someone who is excitable, so long as you discuss in advance the rules. Do not allow her to challenge you or force you to do anything you don't want to do. Make sure she understands that she is the sub, meaning she follows directions, and you are the one dominating her not the other way around.

#62: If you sense the relationship is becoming imbalanced, end it or threaten to end it.

Do not make an idle threat. The sub must understand what she is doing wrong and be given the opportunity to cooperate. If she does not, you must have the strength to end the relationship.

If the sub is very good at persuasion, you may not even realize you are in a bad relationship until several sessions into it. When this happens, it is time to stop the abuse, or if not "abuse" per se, then the one sided relationship that it's becoming.

Do not doubt your own instincts. One of the things that subs are told to ask themselves in aftercare is whether they feel "raped" after a session. The answer, of course, should always be no. But the same is true for the Dom. If you feel as if you have been coerced into doing something you didn't want to do, or if you feel shamed in any way, then it's no longer a productive relationship and it should end.

This may be difficult for you if you are just now gaining experience and this is only your first or second relationship. But the emotional abuse you may endure may not be worth it.

#63: Keep on the lookout for these troubling signs, that show a sub who is railing out control.

- She is self-centered

- Rude or inconsiderate

- Demands all of your time and attention—rather than you giving her what you can afford

- Expects you to drop everything to show attention to her (not playing the part of a sub)

- Is rude to other people in your life; in the BDSM community, or in the real world

- Doesn't obey and seems to beg for punishment; craving abuse, but not listening to the direction

- They have no interest in your personal goals, dreams or desires

- Does not want you to go places or have a life to yourself

- Fights out in public

- Criticizes your friends or family

- Displays racist or sexist attitudes outside of role play

- Compares you to other lovers or Doms she had

- Constantly questioning you in a demeaning manor

- Doesn't accept criticism

- Never takes responsibility for her actions; rationalizes that her work colleagues, friends, family, or former Doms/Subs are to blame for her suffering

The last two items are important to consider. Questioning and negotiating are part of the process and no sub should ever be told that her questions and criticisms are invalid. However, if you notice that the negotiation process is always one-sided, there is a problem.

If the sub never takes your advice, never considers your wisdom or ideas worthy, and is always criticizing your technique then you are in a bad relationship.

This may not necessarily mean that the sub is a psycho (though she usually is) but simply put, you two are not compatible. A relationship in the BDSM lifestyle is like any other. Equal parts negotiation, not just one person making demands and always needing to "win". It's not about bullying the other person into cooperation.

#64: Be on the lookout for subs who may experiencing depression, rage or other manageable personality disorders.

If you sense that the sub is suffering from a personality disorder or state of depression, you have to exercise good judgment. You are not obligated to role play with them, but if you feel you can handle it, it may be beneficial to help them process their grief and hopefully work towards becoming a more well-adjusted person.

People who are on this "downward spiral" tend to exhibit these symptoms:

- They are bouncing job to job, showing household instability

- They disregards laws or social customs

- They are angry about government or religious societies controlling their lives

- Paranoid about being embarrassed in front of others

- Seems to exhibit a different personality when out in public

- Accuse you of keeping secrets or being unfaithful

- Jealous of the attention you receive from other people

- Tries to use guilt or suicidal thoughts as manipulative behavior

- Persists in aggressive or hurtful behavior

- Never apologizes or apologizes and resumes the same conduct

- Shows inconsistency in other life patterns; i.e. sexual relationships

- Over indulges in alcohol, marijuana or sex—the "legal" vices

These relationships will be exhausting and are not recommended for first-time Doms. But if you sincerely want to help these people, you can. Give them the attention they deserve but give it at a price—they must follow your orders and not simply provoke you into their bidding.

#65: Decipher how much punishment/reward a sub gets, based on her personality traits.

Granted, not all subs are "crazy" or mentally unstable. Sometimes they are just dealing with a lot of issues but are fairly normal and just need BDSM play to help them overcome some of their buried issues. They do play well with a Dom, but only if he knows what he's doing. If the Dom is lacking in intelligence or maturity, the sub will only be frustrated. So these are what you might call "advanced" subs that are quite a handful. They can be recognized by these characteristics:

- They are very talkative and talking helps them realize their feelings before they even know how they feel

- They are not self-assured; usually self-conscious and/or nervous

- They don't necessarily do well with sexual tension or social pressure

- They seem to enjoy controversial conversation or shocking statements from Doms or men or others; most well-adjusted people seem to avoid controversial discussions as they find them exhausting or stressful

- They gossip a lot about other people, especially their faults

- Her social activities tend to be passionate but always tentative; her interests and hobbies change quickly; they get bored of the stimulation and move onto something else they can be good at

- She frequently makes friends, who become enemies; she has a revolving door of social acquaintances and drama always seems to come and go

- Her friends consist of people who adore her (very often the case with pretty women) and so she is constantly reassured by others, giving her a bit of an unrealistic view of herself.

- She is very charismatic and sociable, but only with you…she doesn't seem to have a large social network

- They admit to you depression and or other minor personality flaws

- They seem to isolate themselves from crowds

The last two items are interesting, as they are a reminder that much of the population you meet will have issues. There is no "perfect partner" and quite frankly, the lifestyle attracts some people with a variety of neuroses.

Now these characteristics, while intimidating, do not necessarily mean you should stay away. It just means you have to invest serious effort into correcting and disciplining their thinking.

The fact that these subs are often sociable and charismatic is not a bad thing...unless they really don't socialize with people in general. If this is the case, they probably have a history of charming individuals and taking something from them. It may be the sub's own need for attention and validation to help address their uncertainty about themselves.

If you decide to take on a troubled sub, you need to be nurturing but very authoritative. In the next chapter, we're going to discuss ways to create a curriculum that helps heal the wounded ego.

Chapter 11: Creating a Therapeutic Curriculum to Build Self-Esteem

While you may understand that some subs suffer from low self-esteem and other issues, figuring out how to improve their thinking may still be a challenge. It's best that you do NOT improvise or create a plan of action from your own instincts. Instead, follow the structures of real course development and proven psychology.

Let's start by reviewing how professors and teachers develop a traditional curriculum.

#66: Create a curriculum of training in a similar manner to a traditional curriculum; namely these steps:

- Determine the objective in advance (for example, stop a sub from hating herself)

- Create a theme for all your sessions, as well as mantras and thoughts that you want the sub to focus on

- Create a sequence of milestones that the sub must learn that will teach them necessary individual skills that will allow the objective

- Develop a list of punishments and rewards to motivate the sub and make her avoid falling back into old patterns.

- The punishments should not be pleasurable but disappointing or moderately painful in some way (always according to discussed hard/soft limits)

- Create an assessment device, which can help measure the progress of the sub. If she is still lacking in some way, more training may be needed.

- Keep goals measurable and realistic, within a reasonable amount of time/sessions

- Communicate during the negotiation, pre-session and aftercare, regarding the sub's feelings and how they feel about the session.

It might help to explain to the sub how and why they feel the way they do in advance. The sub may already be conscious of the "why" but hearing the lessons again, in advance of training, may help tremendously. One effective technique in this regard is to explain how training works and how we can reprogram ourselves to think differently and act differently.

So your intent is to:

#67: Discuss the changes that the sub will be experiencing and explain how that's going to happen through punishment and reward.

Self-awareness should not be a problem. You are not a magician or even a psychologist. You are training the sub to embrace the "new identity". There's no complicated training needed and no need to hide anything. Help her "feel" what she already knows intellectually. Make her experience unpleasant for wrong thinking or behavior and reward her with good progress.

Part of this unorthodox "therapy" will be helping the sub to relax and meditate on the new personality. This is why touching and calming thoughts from you are so important during the aftercare. You are reinforcing her beliefs and instincts, and all of those should be positive. You are re-teaching her how to love herself.

#68: Use a few tools to engage your sub and draw out her real feelings. Help her uncover something about herself and try to help her understand how she feels.

Some of these visualization tasks include:

- Drawing out her inner child by telling her to draw something abstract. Eventually the "inner child" focuses on the details of the abstract image and draws more details. Spend about twenty minutes on this task and then have her turn the paper over and describe what she drew.

- Have the sub create a future collage, based on their perceived future. Where will she be in 20 years? Determine if her present course needs to change to meet her desires for the future. Since you are piecing together images (or using a site like Pinterest) it's easier to think abstractly and encourage honest thought.

- Have the sub create / describe their outer self and inner self. They can use a literal mask or just use the concept. Have them describe the differences in what they show people, and what they really are inside. Have them think about who they share their inner self with and who sees their outer self.

- Have her write a love letter to herself. Stick to the positives and have them write down encouraging words. It's important to teach subs with low self-esteem to be kind and loving to themselves and not just other people.

- Have the sub paint a self portrait. Get all the painting tools necessary and draw herself in whatever natural way she can. Make the sub spend time thinking about herself and why she drew what she did. Teach her not to judge what she sees but to be honest. Teach her to find beauty and not only flaws.

- Create affirmations. Whether using cards or another multimedia form, write down affirmations that the sub needs to hear, usually what is opposite to her way of pessimistic or self-loathing thinking. Not only do you write down the affirmation but also the image associated with the affirmation. Instruct the sub to keep these affirmations all around her as inspiration throughout the day. This will help in rewiring her natural thoughts.

All of these recommendations are basic training in Cognitive Behavior Therapy, which works to adjust negative thoughts and behaviors associated with negative thoughts. By changing these thoughts into positive thoughts and feelings, behavior can improve.

By now you have the basic tools down to create a plan of BDSM training for your sub. Use your own creativity to develop a learning course and create a limited number of sessions, which you can change later on if necessary. This is another reason why it's important to be compatible with your sub intellectually and emotionally, so that the two of you can work together.

Obviously, you are limited in what you can do as you are not a doctor or therapist. A Dom is not a replacement for serious mental disorders or potentially harmful behavior. The next chapter will discuss how to handle subs who are beyond your control and dangerous.

Chapter 12: Getting Professional Involved

There's not much to say about getting your sub the professional help she needs. It isn't your job; it isn't what you're trained for; and you don't want to put yourself in a position of accountability if they should bottom out or worse. Don't take on more responsibility than you can handle. You don't even have to take a sub under your wing if you feel uncomfortable.

#69: You CAN offer guidance but you cannot offer professional therapy unless you are trained in that.

Professional therapy from a licensed professional focuses on precisely what to say to stop a person from killing or harming themselves, or how to help them conquer addiction with physical help. Much of the process involves teaching them coping mechanisms. BDSM sessions with you are not a legitimate coping mechanism—just the preliminary step to creating a new mindset.

So while you can do a lot of good for a sub and direct her in the right direction, it does not serve your best interest or hers to replace a doctor's treatment.

Furthermore, sending your sub to a therapist or doctor is going to protect you from litigation should anything major happen to the poor girl.

This brings up a point…should you have sex or "play" with someone who's mentally or emotionally suffering?

#70: Decide in advance what you can afford to lose and what she can afford to lose.

Do not enter a relationship because you think you can save her. Only enter in if you believe you can help and she is mentally capable of understanding that you're helping her.

This means that:

1. You do not take on subs who are going to end up hurting you or costing you too much of your time, your heart or your resources.

2. You do not take on a sub that IMMEDIATELY needs medical attention, such as someone dying from drug addiction or someone that is suicidal or homicidal. In this case, it's best to stage an intervention with their family. Do not put yourself in a compromising situation with someone who is dangerous.

3. A Dom does not want to save a sub, unless he wants a full-time slave. A Dom wants to HELP a sub get back on her feet, as in a temporary assignment.

4. Lastly, determine whether the sub has the intellectual capacity and maturity to understand how you are helping them. If you sense that they are not all there mentally or emotionally, then do not offer them assistance.

The reason for (4) being, that a psychopathic sub is really your worst nightmare. If she suddenly decides she's not happy with you, she can make your life miserable. She could stalk you, claim you raped her or took advantage of her sexually when she was feeling vulnerable.

Once again, if she lacks the intelligence, maturity and real knowledge of the BDSM community and its high standards, do not get involved.

#71: When telling a sub to go for professional treatment, direct her to a specific place and not just "in general."

A sub is much like a child in that she does not figure out what to do unless you direct her. Assuming that she is emotionally stable enough to have a relationship with, but still suffers from depression or some kind of downward spiral (like dangerous sexual conduct which is quite common) then at some point you might want to recommend attending professional therapy as a means of bettering herself.

Choose a specific doctor or therapist. Direct her where to go and make the decision for her. She will usually follow through, provided that you address her concerns and gradually build up to this goal. Do not surprise her with it and do not "force" her to do it. You are simply recommending it to her as a task that will earn a reward.

#72: You do not have to stop seeing the sub while therapy goes on.

The only reason you stop seeing the sub is if the relationship comes to an end or if she is emotionally unbalanced to the point of danger. However, if she is still safe and sane and willing to experiment with you, then by all means keep disciplining her and rewarding her while she seeks the professional help she needs.

You may be the temporary motivation for her while she re-learns new coping mechanisms in her life. If this is the case, then reward her for doing as she asks and seeks help from a therapist.

#73: Rather than approach the situation as a punishment, approach it in a positive light. You want your sub to do this so she can better herself, to better please you.

Simply telling the sub that she's pathetic and needs to see a doctor is a terrible blow to her self-esteem. So take a positive note with it. Tell her that you want to see her improve in her self-esteem. Tell her that the therapist can help her to cope better, to become a better sub, and to please you the way you need to be pleased.

While naturally, this is all for her benefit, she might enjoy the illusion that this is part of the BDSM game or session. She doesn't want to admit that she's suffering or mentally disturbed. That's negative. Put a positive slant on it and she will be more willing to cooperate. Just be sure to reward her well for taking such a huge positive step in her life.

You as the Dom are your sub's motivation. If you can help her towards a goal of better mental health, and seeking professional help, you have done this person a very wonderful service.

A sub can definitely be a handful…but have you ever considered handling multiple subs? That's quite a challenge and that's the focus of our next few chapters.

Chapter 13: Working with Multiple Subs and Other Doms

Of course, having multiple partners as a sub or Dom is complex...but honestly, having multiple partners is one reason why many get into the alternative lifestyles. Learning such a hierarchy is necessary so that you can minimize hurt feelings, angry friends or acquaintances and socially awkward misunderstandings.

The first thing to realize is that there has to be some order to such "freedom" or else it would be sexual chaos. We've already reviewed some of the standards we strive to keep when dealing with individuals one on one. Now it's time to discuss some of the more complex motivations and standards we need to adhere by when playing with multiple partners, either Doms or subs.

#74: Understand that there are different strokes for different folks!

Quite literally in the BDSM world. Some Doms may be satisfied with having just one sub. However, other Doms may want to own multiple subs. So as long as the subs know about each other there is usually no problem. Unlike say, polygamy, these relationships are all based on the idea of willful submission and the freedom to walk away at any time. Therefore there is far more tolerance in the BDSM community as regards having multiple friends or even lovers within the lifestyle. There is no infidelity when consent and knowledge is shared.

#75: Realistically speaking, subs must be given permission by a Dom to have multiple Doms.

There has to be an alpha Dom at some point that has final control over the sub. He may allow the sub to see other people but he has to determine, along with the sub's input, just how these other Doms are going to train the sub. Will the training be in conflict to the original Dom's criteria? If so, this would be a negative relationship that would hurt the original one.

The original Dom also has to decide if the sub is ready to have multiple Doms and if these other Doms are qualified to dispense training or if they are of poor quality.

Therefore, in theory the sub starts with one Dom and then earns the right to see other Doms when the alpha Dom sees that there is room for improvement with multiple "teachers." A sub that just chooses to see any Dom she wants will probably receive conflicting messages and start a disruption, if not in the community itself, then at least inside her own head.

#76: Understand that not just one Dom can complete one sub, or vice versa.

Since BDSM practice tends to be hyper-focused in one area, it is quite possible that a sub will need multiple Doms to get the complete experience, as will Doms need more than one sub to feel fully valued in the community.

Some Doms can only provide limited training, especially if they avoid sexual relations. A sub might find it advantageous to have a number of Doms for different purposes; such as, healing, masochism, and so on.

Switches play both sub and Dom are also have more complex issues to deal with, and may benefit from having multiple partners. In any event close communication is necessary, with the sub and Dom, and the sub and the other Dom. There cannot be scheduling conflicts or else that can lead to neglect or disrespectful conduct.

Ideally, the two Doms would communicate to make sure each other's curriculum is balanced. If this is not possible, then the sub should definitely make an effort to honestly convey the information to both Doms so that a schedule can be figured out.

Remember that some Doms excel in certain areas but not others. There may be Doms who are dominant in bed but not in other areas of life where a sub desires attention. Some Doms may be gay, bisexual or heterosexual. Some may not have sex with any of their subs but may offer spankings, training, hypnosis, and so on.

In general, if a sub is collared she is owned and so she reports to her original Dom. She must receive permission from him and usually in person if she wants to be trained by others.

Speaking of which…

#77: A Dom should not keep a harem of slaves if he doesn't have the time to devote to all of them.

Frankly it's unrealistic for a Dom to have six or seven subs as it's hard to imagine having the time to adequately train all of them. If an orgy is desired that's a lot more practical in terms of time than actually owning a few subs and having to make curriculum for every one of them.

A Dom should only keep as many subs as he can train and has the resources to train. Otherwise, he is not being a good Dom and subs would find no particular reason to work with him.

But what happens when two Doms start fighting?

#78: Multiple Doms training a sub have to cooperate.

Two or more Doms simply have to collaborate so as not to confuse the sub. In the worst case scenario, the Doms may even fight over the sub and the sub will have to choose one over the other. In these cases the original Dom or the "Master" is the one who the sub obeys and will stop seeing the other Dom. There does have to be a primary relationship where the sub gives full loyalty.

Nothing is written in stone and there probably have been rebellious subs that have dumped their Dom for another Dom. But the ideal is always cooperation.

Live In Situations and Ownership

What oftentimes happens is that the sub falls in love with the Dom, or both fall in love at the same time and simply cannot stop seeing each other. While this is certainly a different type of love than the usual romantic monogamous relationship, the dynamic is similar. It is even similar to a traditional monotheistic religious marriage, where the man (or in this case the Dom/ Domme) exercises headship over the household.

The sub who has been trained to the extent that she cannot leave the Dom has become a "slave," though it's possible the Dom will choose another name. The slave is a lifetime committed sub, who has assumed a subservient role to the Dom, or "Master." While it's true that the slave is always free to go at any time, the idea is that she doesn't want to leave and would rather pledge loyalty for the rest of her life and his life.

#79: Giving your sub the role of a slave accomplishes two things: it keeps the relationship indefinite and ongoing and it also opens up your relationship to experimenting with other partners.

You may choose to mark your sub with a collar or with a tattoo or something else physical that demonstrates "ownership" of the sub for an indefinite period of time. The sub enjoys the feeling of being owned, protected and watched out for. It is not a matter of shame and any Dom who would put a collar or mark on a sub, without request, is not a real Dom.

#80: Multiple slaves owned by the same Dom will cooperate with one another and assume a family situation. They will watch out for one another and figure out ways to cooperate.

These slaves usually want a Master with similar characteristics and so they are willing to be led by one and to share him with other subs, rather than settle for a Dom who isn't that talented at what he does.

They may find it advantageous to move into the same house. So you may occasionally see ads for a Dom and his slaves looking for another sub or slave. This is not always as easy a situation as it seems. There are standards and protocols you have to learn in order to live peacefully with the other subs and the Dom. These relationships also tend to be short-lived, because frankly it's hard to find subs that are willing to grow into the role of slaves in a group environment. The communication is not as intimate.

This has given credence to the idea that:

#81: Doms controls subs for a limited span of time. Masters own slaves indefinitely.

When you try to break the laws or standards of this simple line of reasoning, problems ensue. You cannot expect a new sub to act like a slave. You cannot expect a slave to be treated as casually as a new sub because there are family bonds here.

All slaves desire great and exclusive attention. Subs also need attention and reassurance and not planning these activities in advance can be disastrous.

Managing Subs and Giving Them All Something to Do

First determine if you want a group setting, where there is one Dom controlling multiple subs or if multiple Doms control multiple slaves. You may occasionally see the latter at High Protocol BDSM parties, where one Dom / Master allows others to enjoy his slave in a limited capacity.

#82: The goal is to decide in advance what each sub will be doing and WHY.

If each sub has a goal and has an understanding of her task, then the operation will go smoothly and resemble a work environment. Each "employee" must know and understand his task so as to prevent conflict with other employees. The same dynamic is true when a Dom is juggling a few subs.

Are you just lazily telling them to make love to you at once? Or are you giving them a task that fits hand in hand with their individual training? A Dom must take the multiple sub scenario very seriously and make an effort to plan everything—leaving no one feeling neglected.

A few subs may be showing difficulty in one area and if that's the case, having fun with multiple subs might not be a good idea—not if the Dom is clueless about how to resolve their individual problems in a group setting.

On the other hand, if the Dom decides that one sub is shy and needs experience doing sexual things in front of other men or women, they might find it useful to expose the sub to a group setting. There must be a reason for every action you take. A sub's life is not to be toyed with.

#83: Teach the subs not to contradict anything that their Dom tells them, whether that's you or someone else.

It is the first priority of the lifestyle that the sub obeys the Dom, so as long as the submission protocol is proper. Therefore the Dom would make it a point to work with other Doms and acknowledge the ownerships of certain subs.

He would not issue any orders that he knew would violate the sub's protocol with another Dom. This spirit of camaraderie will also ensure that the subs look out for each other, and the Doms look out for each other.

They will help enforce rules and punishments and improve communication.

#84: Before going to an event, make sure the sub knows who the acting Dom is for a specific period of time.

This doesn't mean that other Doms should be ignored or that the sub can't play with another Dom. It simply means that one Dom has the final say. This is what will keep the event organized. And no one will be stealing from someone else.

#85: Be kind to other Doms!

You may oftentimes run into other Doms. And there is certainly no reason to be cold or even "dominant" to other Doms. They are your allies. And if you work well together, you could even borrow each other's subs. Do not take the same tone that you take with a sub when you are talking to a Dom. Doms have equal respect among each other.

Of course, this doesn't mean you should be sheepish or overly deferring. That will very quickly paint you as a weak Dom. You do want to appear confident, in control and knowledgeable, but with the capacity to be kind to your fellow Doms and their subs.

Remember that no one is "better" than anyone else in the BDSM world. We all have roles to play and understanding those roles comes mutual respect. We don't compare partners or subs or Doms. We remain positive and always eager to learn and teach each other.

In the next chapter, we're going to learn more about troubleshooting multiple subs or Doms.

Chapter 14: Dealing with Jealousy or Rivalries

Subs seem to have more jealousy issues than Doms do, though there certainly have been Dom Wars within the BDSM community. When troubleshooting strained relationships, it's important to avoid getting ego involved and certainly no macho "you do what I say!" crap.

The best way to handle real life jealousy is to analyze the problem objectively and especially when out of character.

#86: Determine the difference between jealousy and envy.

Jealousy is a fear and oftentimes a weakness. It is a malfunction and a problem that needs to be carefully analyzed and addressed.

Envy is pretty easy to solve. You give the neglected sub what she wants, that the other sub already has, but what the envious sub is lacking.

#87: Since jealousy involves the fear of losing what you already have, the goal is to spend more time with the jealous sub assuring her that nothing is going to change.

Right now she lacks trust and a feeling of security. Jealousy is the symptom of the problem, not the problem itself. Spending a little more time reassuring her and rewarding her is the best way to handle this. Do NOT punish her as the opposite treatment for such weakness is aggression.

In addition to reassurance…

#88: Find additional causes by opening a sincere line of communication.

This should be out of character and you should broach every subject imaginable even if it seems unrelated. All of the sub's emotions are valid and they must understand how seriously you take this obligation to watch and protect them.

#89: Adjust your curriculum of training to make more time and more sessions to overcoming the sub's new fear.

Jealousy will soon dissipate once the sub realizes that trust and security are at an all-time high. The goal in these sessions and in the aftercare conversation is to discuss the root of the jealousy and where the fear comes from. What can the Dom and sub do to address these fears and improve the general mood of the sub? Making necessary changes is the next logical step.

#90: Once practical changes are made to accommodate the sub, the sub must learn to control her jealousy.

If she feels jealousy on an instinctive level then help her to learn how to transform jealousy to a more rational emotion. In other words, you teach her how to deal with these feelings, in addition to treating her for the root cause.

Always be a good listener. And communicate with respect, never with anger, so that the sub is encouraged to open her heart.

#91: When a sub is envious, determine when and where the best time is to give the sub what she desires.

Don't just cave in and give her what she wants. You have to determine if she's ready for it and when a proper time frame is for allowing her to experience it. It's best to actually create a series of events getting gradually closer to what she envies, rather than simply pouring it on her just because she wants it.

#92: You can be proactive and actually test the jealousy of your sub when you think she's ready for it…and only if it fits into your self-improvement curriculum.

Testing the sub's limits as regards self-confidence and jealousy/envy is a good idea, as you can anticipate problems she might have in the future. Even if your sub doesn't indicate jealousy or insecurity, it would be wise to see if these are issues that might come up months after your sessions finally end.

#93: Remember that your sub is part of your own reputation. If you do a negligent job, your sub will badmouth you.

Or even if she doesn't, people who know her will ask about who trained her. If you are negligent you will be unleashing a sub to a world which she isn't equipped to deal with.

Now you see how important it is to spend adequate time training each sub?

How to Keep Multiple Subs Safe and Happy

If a rivalry is starting between subs that you own/supervise, then obviously the best thing to do is to separate them. Do not let subs that resent each other work together. This may be somewhat standard in other teaching venues, but in BDSM it's not really conducive to a good scene.

Instead…

#94: Spend time with each sub individually and help them control their jealousy or envy.

When they can understand the root of their jealousy, then they might be able to play nice again. However, if you sense that the sub just wants to drain your energy and keeps going over the same things over and over again, it's better to just let her go. Some subs just like draining their Masters / Doms and have no real interest in changing. You always have a choice to move on if you've tried your best.

And yes, if you have a bad experience with a sub, from her end, you can tell others in the BDSM community to beware of her.

#95: If you have rivalries between subs that involve other Doms then make it a point to always talk to the other Master / Dom first.

Just out of basic respect, you don't approach subs with requests unless their Dom lets them. Perhaps you can get the other Dom to help in her jealousy training.

However, if this doesn't help, then you may simply have to choose one sub over another. If one sub is forcing you to choose, manipulating your behavior, this could be signs of an unstable or mentally ill sub, since this is not the proper role for a sub.

At the end of the day, you must make tough choices and this involves putting your sub's protection above your own interest. If a sub cannot handle working with another sub you must choose to either separate them, or end one relationship in hopes of keeping another productive.

Naturally, when engaging in safe and consensual BDSM play, always make sure that when engaging in polyamorous relationships, that everybody is regularly tested for STIs and that everyone leaves **happily**.

If your sub is not happy or if the relationship is not well, do not just abandon the sub if at all possible. (Unless of course she's insane and you fear for your life) Whenever you can, help her find another Dom who can better address her needs.

What if you're eager to fulfill your fantasy and hers and introduce multiple participants in one scene? Let's get kinky in the next chapter.

Chapter 15: Parties, Threesomes, and Orgies with Multiple Subs

The good news (well if you're engaging in an orgy that IS the good news) is that there are only a few very simple rules when it comes to playing with multiple subs and Doms.

#96: When you're a guest be respectful and pay attention to the rules.

#97: When planning a party of your own, spend time making rules and making sure your guests are protected and have fun.

When it comes to being a guest, the rules will usually be posted on the invitation or at the party itself. The following sets of rules are standard etiquette whether you're hosting or attending and they involve common courtesy.

#98: Be conscientious of other Doms and subs by following basic sex etiquette:

- Always bringing condoms and lubricant.
- Always arriving clean, showered and smelling nice (But be careful about heavily scented perfume/cologne).
- Groom according to the standards of the party. (For instance they usually ask men to shave).
- Wear high quality clothing, including undergarments
- If you have open wounds, do not attend.
- Adhering to the dress code.
- Bring rubber gloves, sanitizing wipes, soap and towels.
- Do not attend if you're sick!
- Do not break the rules under any circumstances.

The rules will always be posted and in some cases you may even have to sign a waiver indicating consent that you will follow instructions.

#99: If you are bringing subs you must ensure they follow the rules as well because they represent you and your reputation.

Determine in advance what you and your subs' boundaries are. You do NOT have to submit to the rules of other Doms or the "house" if they are in violation of your own boundaries. If that's the case just leave.

Most of these events take your comfort very seriously so as long as you communicate with your subs all should be well. Be sure to create a safe word for your subs in case any of them panic and need protection later in the evening.

#100: Go to the room you will be most comfortable with and follow the directions of the acting Dom.

Most large events have different rooms for different kinks. You may even find that orgy events have a room for BDSM, and other rooms for touching, kissing, dancing, swinger sex and so on.

Usually a Dom will be directing the scene and managing the toys; for instance, chains, whips, floggers, gadgets and so on. The Dom is not just having fun—his job is to supervise the party to make sure no one gets hurt and everyone has fun. So show respect and follow his lead.

#101: Do not start with "in character" talks. Have normal conversations at first and be friendly. Once you are accepted into a scene you can start speaking in character.

Act like a normal person. Be confident but be polite and in a good mood. Make sure your subs are also enjoying themselves. Your subs should be well behaved. Having to discipline your subs in public would be a bit embarrassing for both of you. Be aware that many people will use aliases instead of their real name during events like these.

#102: Always be positive. Compliment people, since everyone is a little self-conscious at sexually themed events.

Don't be negative. Be supportive. While you won't feel attracted to everyone, there's always a reason to be polite and encouraging to everyone at the event. In fact, the sooner you begin complimenting others on their outfit or their body, the sooner you might get an invitation to participate.

#103: Be inclusive and think about your subs.

Sometimes you may be invited to participate as a Dom, but your sub might get dismissed. If the sub is okay with that, you can work with it. But if your sub is jealous then do consider her feelings. It is somewhat disrespectful to exclude someone. You can always ask if your sub(s) can take part in the scene too. If not, you always have a choice to say "No thanks. I only play as a team."

#104: Never just "do." Ask for consent.

This is not only polite but it also protects you. Always get consent, in the form of a question. Do not simply walk up and start playing with a person, even if they smile. It's just good etiquette to ask first.

The questioning phase is a part of BDSM activity anyway and just because this is an unusual environment doesn't mean it's not needed. Asking and answering questions can be erotic so have fun with it and don't underestimate the importance.

#105: Don't take rejection personally.

Orgies would be out of control if everybody said yes to everybody. So don't take rejection of you or your sub personally. Remember that some people only like to watch or only like to play with their own sub/Dom. They may not want activity with anyone they don't know. So focus on making friends first and watching others have fun.

If you are invited, take it as a compliment. Play with your own sub and give everyone else a show to watch. Maybe the next party you will get the invitation you've been waiting for.

Instructing Multiple Subs in a Sex Scene

It can be clumsy to direct three or four different people in a sex scene. The key to hosting a successful encounter involving more than two people is to…

#106: Make sure everyone has something to do at all times.

One sub being left out and bored is the worst scenario possible. Therefore, give each sub specific instruction, whether it's to help pleasure the Dom or pleasure another sub.

You don't have to choreograph the scene in great detail. Simply instruct the sub to follow you through movement. Show the other sub how you want them to use their hands or lips and then move on to the next sub.

#107: Since you are the Dom you must take the lead in showing subs how you want to be pleasured, and then factor in how best to pleasure each sub.

You may have to take turns with pleasuring one sub, using the other sub, but don't stop the scene until everyone's had their turn for maximum pleasure. You must take the lead in showing the subs how to pleasure you. But you must also be smart and know what the subs want to experience selfishly and how multiple lovers can enhance that experience.

#108: If you get two subs working together and pleasuring each other, do not interrupt the flow of energy. Let them build to a peak of excitement and release before changing the position or scene.

Finish a thought, basically. If you keep interrupting a scene, just when an orgasm is imminent you might inadvertently frustrate the sub. In general, threesomes tend to leave one partner by himself, at least momentarily, so be proactive in finding something to do as the Dom, whether it's just playing with yourself or caressing or kissing the bodies of your busy subs.

This may take practice but after a few sessions you will get the hang of it.

#109: When staging your own event for visitors, use your imagination to make the night memorable.

Creativity and sex always go hand in hand. Have a theme for your orgy or BDSM High Protocol Event.

Try to match your desires and your sub's desires with what some in the community find arousing. Naturally, if you have a very niche specific kink, not all the local populace will find it interesting. But if you widen the location radius, you may find more niche kinksters willing to travel to come enjoy a night.

You could create a list of fetishes and activities you and your subs like and then develop a theme for it, such as "Eyes Wide Shut" night, where everyone wears a masks, or "Fifty Shades" night, where everyone takes turns spanking a sub.

#110: Once you decide upon a fun theme, create your ground rules.

The more rules the better, so as to prevent misunderstandings and to protect all of your guests. Decide on clothing codes, what sex games will be available, what your limits are, and what limits on the guests' behavior will be.

In general, you should ban people from bringing phones or cameras because you don't want these photos getting out!

#111: Create a welcoming and high-end atmosphere.

This means renting a room (or using your own home if you wish) and making it look nice. Think about investing in décor or renting a furniture or toys that are conducive to BDSM activities. Adjoining hotel rooms are a good bet, as they provide plenty of space, as well as room for drinks and refreshments.

Have a public exhibition room, a private room and a "downtime" room just for socializing. Keep condoms stocked, as well as lube, and make sure all toys have new batteries installed. You could have porn videos playing to help get guests in the mood, though the exhibitions are usually far more interesting for guests to watch.

#112: It is advisable to invite BDSM lifestyle compatible members and not random people from Craigslist or Tinder.

While these websites do have plenty of interested attendees, it's simply harder to screen people you haven't met already. This is why finding friends first is a better idea than taking chances.

#113: Don't serve high-alcohol content drinks.

That may seem confusing but think about it. Drunken people don't have fun sex—they cause terrible scenes. They become boisterous, violent and impossible to deal with. It's better that you ask a drunkard to leave rather than risk killing the life of the party.

Besides that, people who are drunk can only give questionable consent. Don't risk someone accusing you of rape just because you were afraid to hurt someone's feelings by sending them home.

Conclusion

We hope you enjoyed some of the more advanced pointers and tidbits that can help you improve your craft. Remember that you have a great opportunity now that you are skilled in Discipline, BDSM play, and role playing. You're not just a good lover or an authority figure…you are a good friend that can help a person come to terms with their demons, get the closure they need, and experience a transformation in their way of thinking.

Being a good Dom is not just naughty fun…it's an art and science if you want to go the extra mile. Don't stop learning. Don't stop helping others. Make yourself available to those in need and you may be surprised at how fulfilling your work in the lifestyle starts to feel.

Other Books by Matthew Larocco

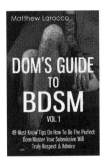
Dom's Guide To BDSM Vol. 1: 49 Must-Know Tips On How To Be The Perfect Dom/Master Your Submissive Will Truly Respect & Admire

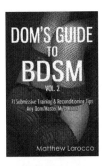
Dom's Guide To BDSM Vol. 2: 71 Submissive Training & Reconditioning Tips Any Dom/Master Must Know

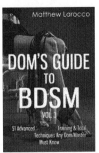
Dom's Guide To BDSM Vol. 3: 51 Advanced Submissive Training & Total Dominance Techniques Any Dom/Master Must Know

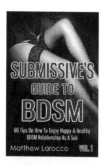
Submissive's Guide To BDSM Vol. 1: 66 Tips On How To Enjoy Happy & Healthy BDSM Relationship As A Sub

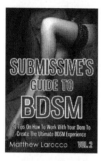
Submissive's Guide To BDSM Vol. 2: 97 Tips On How To Work With Your Dom To Create The Ultimate BDSM Experience

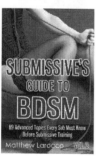
Submissive's Guide To BDSM Vol. 3: 89 Advanced Topics Every Sub Must Know Before Submissive Training

Made in the USA
Columbia, SC
10 December 2021